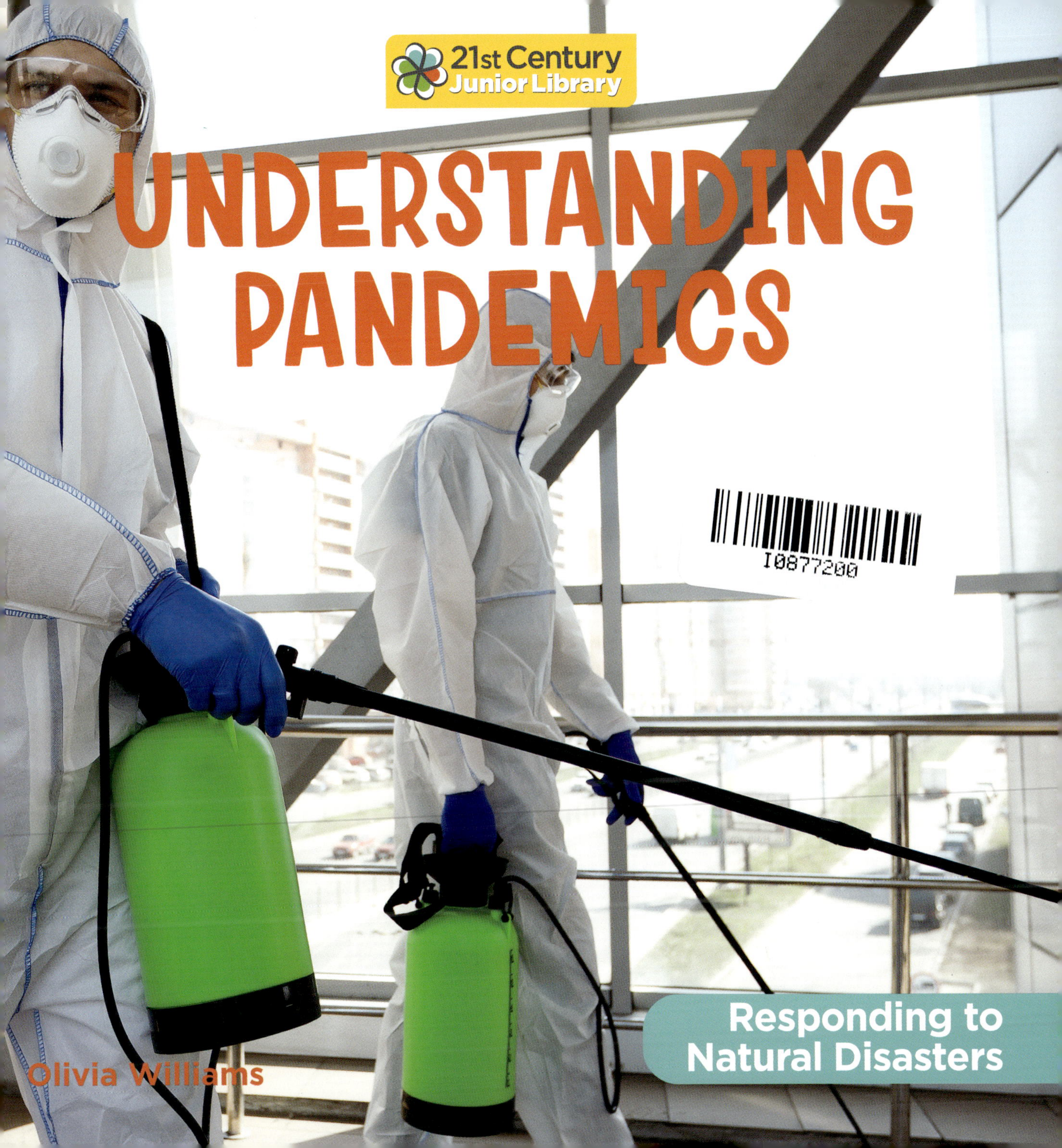

21st Century Junior Library

UNDERSTANDING PANDEMICS

Responding to Natural Disasters

Olivia Williams

Published in the United States of America by:

CHERRY LAKE PRESS
2395 South Huron Parkway, Suite 200, Ann Arbor, Michigan 48104
www.cherrylakepress.com

Reading Adviser: Beth Walker Gambro, MS, Ed., Reading Consultant, Yorkville, IL
Photo Credits: © Prostock-studio/Shutterstock.com, cover, 1; © MVelishchuk/Shutterstock.com, 5; © Rido/Shutterstock.com, 6; © Katya_Bogomolova/Shutterstock.com, 7; © maimoon/Shutterstock.com, 9; © CHOKCHAI POOMICHAIYA/Shutterstock.com, 10, 11; © rchat/Shutterstock.com, 12 [left]; © Ivan Marc/Shutterstock.com, 12 [right]; © engagestock/Shutterstock.com, 13 [top]; © JGA/Shutterstock.com, 13 [bottom, left]; © Efired/Shutterstock.com, 13 [bottom, right]; © TAUFIK ARDIANSYAH/Shutterstock.com, 15 [top]; © Henner Damke/Shutterstock.com, 15 [bottom]; © Diana Taliun/Shutterstock.com, 16; © askarim/Shutterstock.com, 19; © creativeneko/Shutterstock.com, 20; © AnnaStills/Shutterstock.com, 21

Cherry Lake Press is an imprint of Cherry Lake Publishing Group.

Library of Congress Cataloging-in-Publication Data
Names: Williams, Olivia (Writer of children's books), author.
Title: Understanding pandemics / Olivia Williams.
Description: Ann Arbor, MI : Cherry Lake Publishing, [2022] | Series: Responding to natural disasters | Audience: Grades 2-3
Identifiers: LCCN 2021043072 | ISBN 9781534199224 (hardcover) | ISBN 9781668900369 (paperback) | ISBN 9781668901809 (pdf) | ISBN 9781668906125 (ebook)
Subjects: LCSH: Epidemics—Juvenile literature. | Communicable diseases—Juvenile literature.
Classification: LCC RA653.5 .W54 2022 | DDC 614.4—dc23
LC record available at https://lccn.loc.gov/2021043072

Cherry Lake Press would like to acknowledge the work of the Partnership for 21st Century Learning, a Network of Battelle for Kids. Please visit http://www.battelleforkids.org/networks/p21 for more information.

Printed in the United States of America
Corporate Graphics

ABOUT THE AUTHOR

Dr. Olivia Williams is from mid-Wales in the United Kingdom. She has traveled to many countries to help people after natural disasters. She has felt earthquakes and aftershocks, and seen damage from floods, typhoons, and wildfires. The natural environment can be harsh but also beautiful. Olivia loves to hike and run in the mountains and photograph the incredible things she sees.

CHERRY LAKE PRESS

CONTENTS

WHAT ARE PANDEMICS?

A pandemic is a **natural disaster**. It occurs when a new disease quickly spreads around the world. Pandemics usually begin by disease spreading from animals to humans. Scientists quickly try to figure out which country and animal the disease came from. The most recent pandemic is due to a coronavirus, also known as COVID-19. It began in Wuhan, China, in 2019. Like the viruses that have caused other pandemics, COVID-19 is **contagious**.

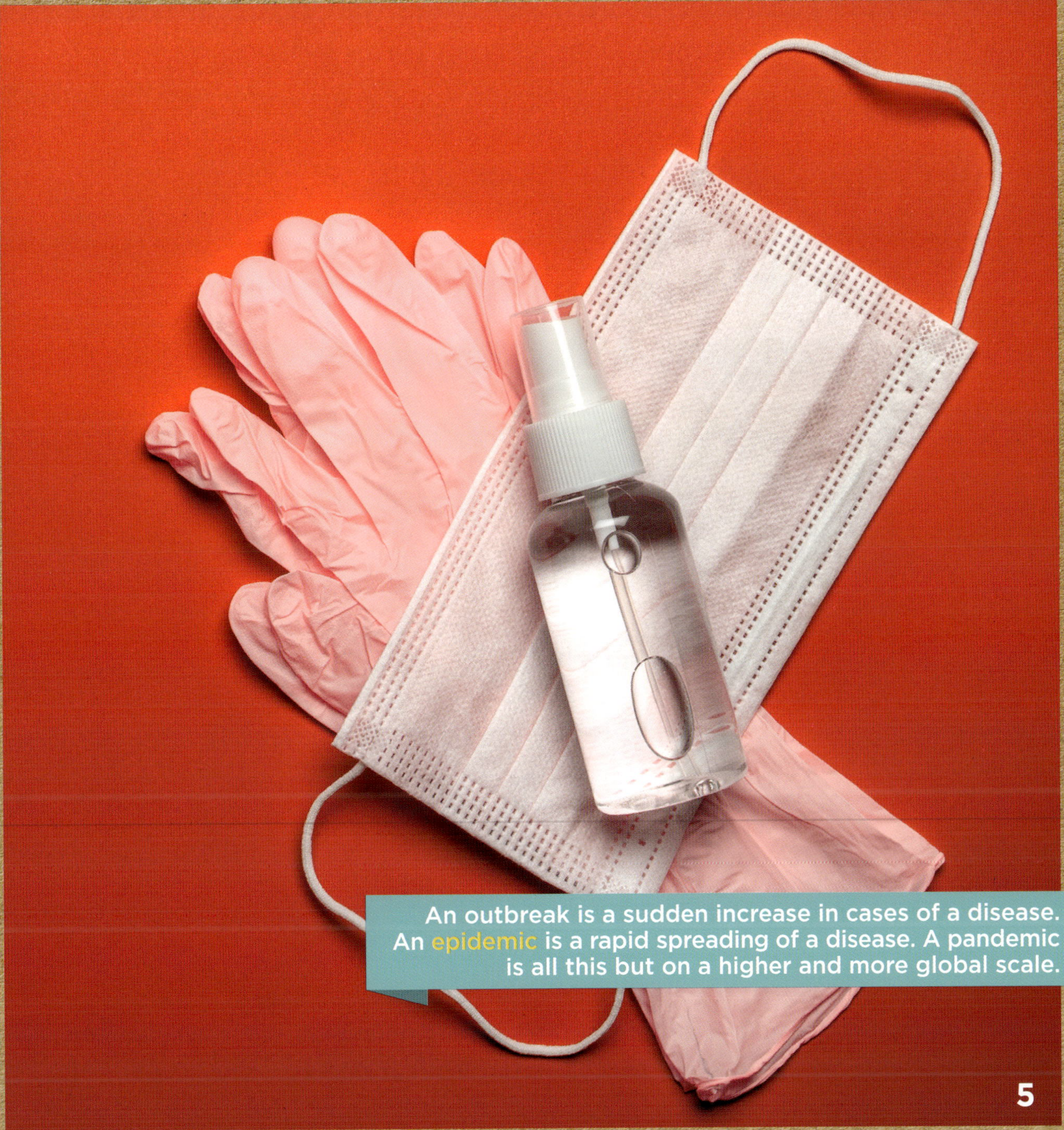

An outbreak is a sudden increase in cases of a disease. An epidemic is a rapid spreading of a disease. A pandemic is all this but on a higher and more global scale.

Pandemics have been happening for hundreds of years. Nearly 700 years ago, a disease spread from Asia to Europe. The disease was called the bubonic plague. Historians think it may have killed as many as 200 million people!

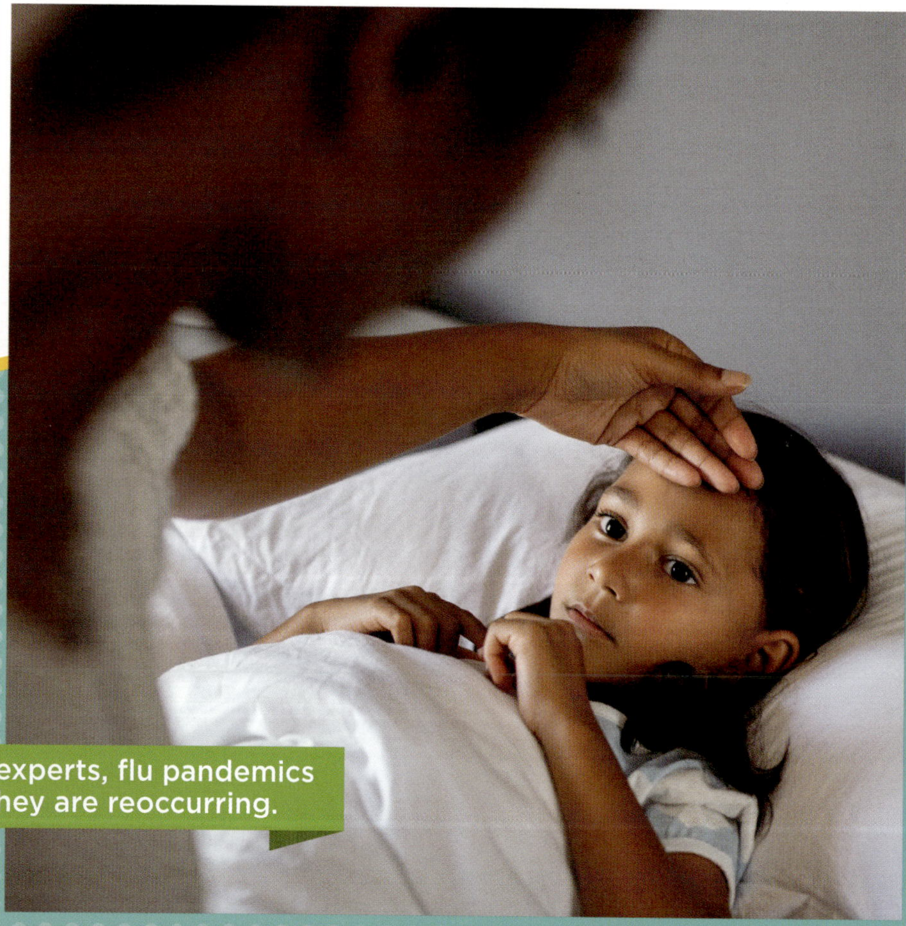

According to experts, flu pandemics are rare, but they are reoccurring.

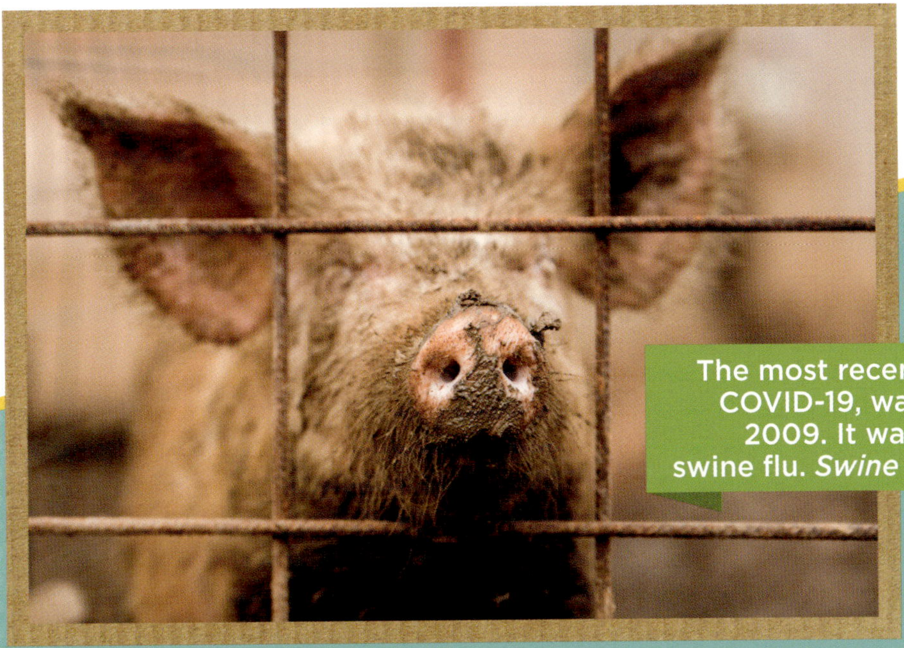

The most recent pandemic, other than COVID-19, was the H1N1 pandemic of 2009. It was also referred to as the swine flu. *Swine* is another word for pig.

The disease traveled fast. It started with infected fleas. These fleas traveled on the backs of rats. The rats lived alongside humans aboard ships. The fleas jumped from rats to humans and bit them, infecting them with the disease. Influenza is another deadly disease. It is commonly known as the flu. The flu affected the world in 1918 and 1919.

It killed 50 million people. It was first identified in birds and pigs.

Cholera was a pandemic that began in 1817 in India. Water and food can contain cholera **bacteria**. People get the illness when the bacteria enter their bodies. Cholera makes people very **dehydrated**. This condition is dangerous and can kill people. Scientists believe that as many as 4 million people are infected with cholera each year. About 143,000 of these infected people die. Communities experiencing poverty are most commonly affected.

Make a Guess!

Before the internet, it would have been difficult to access real-time information about a pandemic. Some people in developing countries still can't access the internet. How do you think we can ensure that people without this access get the information they need?

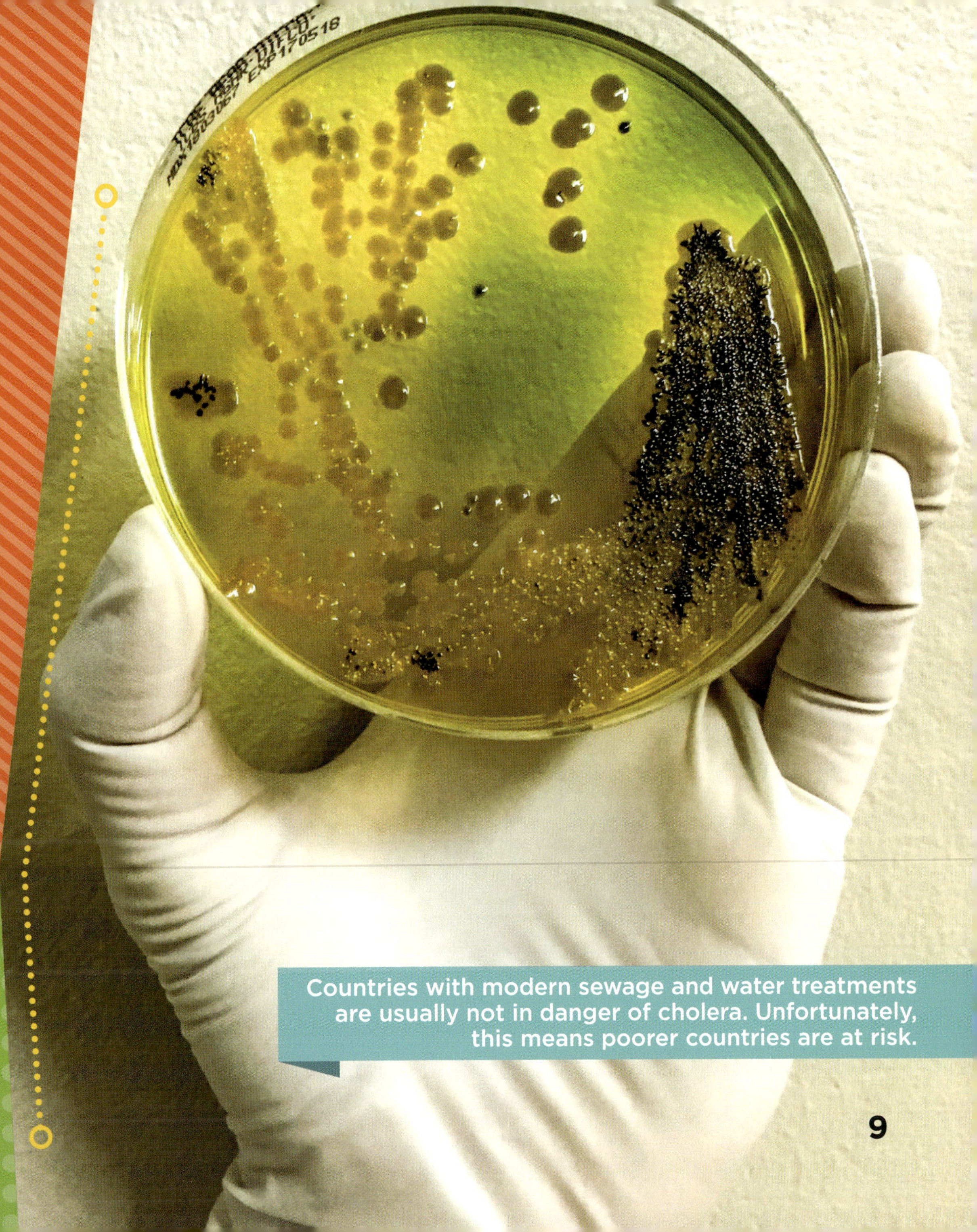

Countries with modern sewage and water treatments are usually not in danger of cholera. Unfortunately, this means poorer countries are at risk.

HOW PANDEMICS AFFECT THE PLANET AND PEOPLE

Generally, the more people who have a disease, the faster it spreads. This is how epidemics become pandemics. Pandemic diseases affect people in different ways. Some people don't have enough natural **immunity**. Their bodies struggle to fight off disease. Some races and ethnicities are more affected than others. This is not due to anything biological. It is related to their **socioeconomic** status.

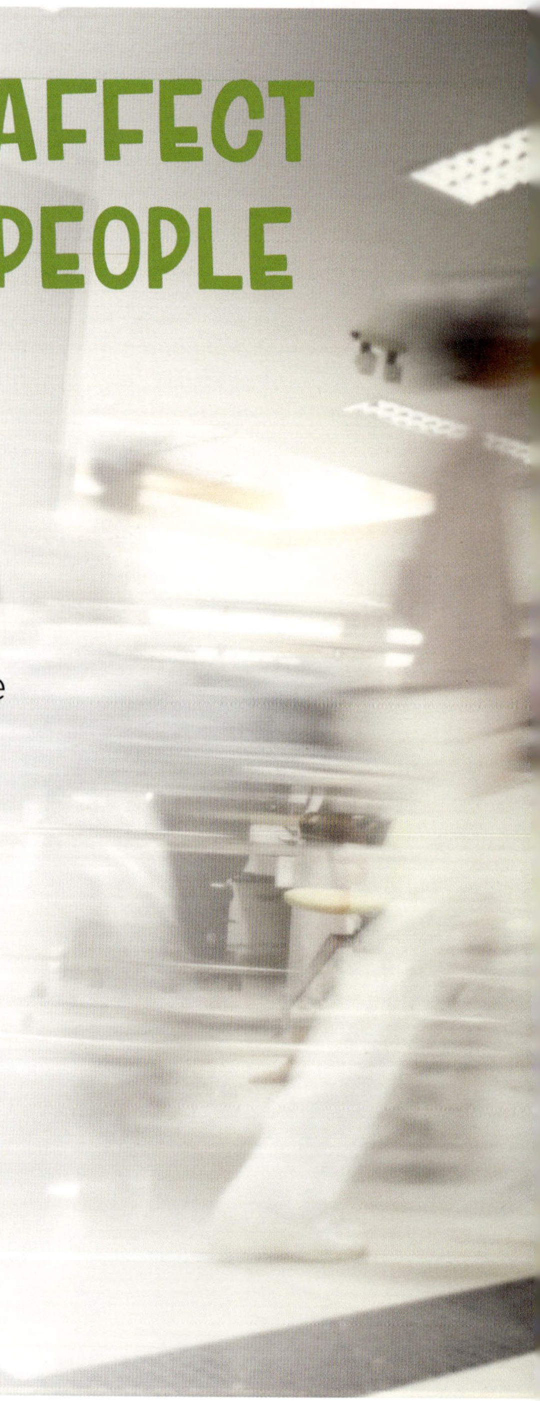

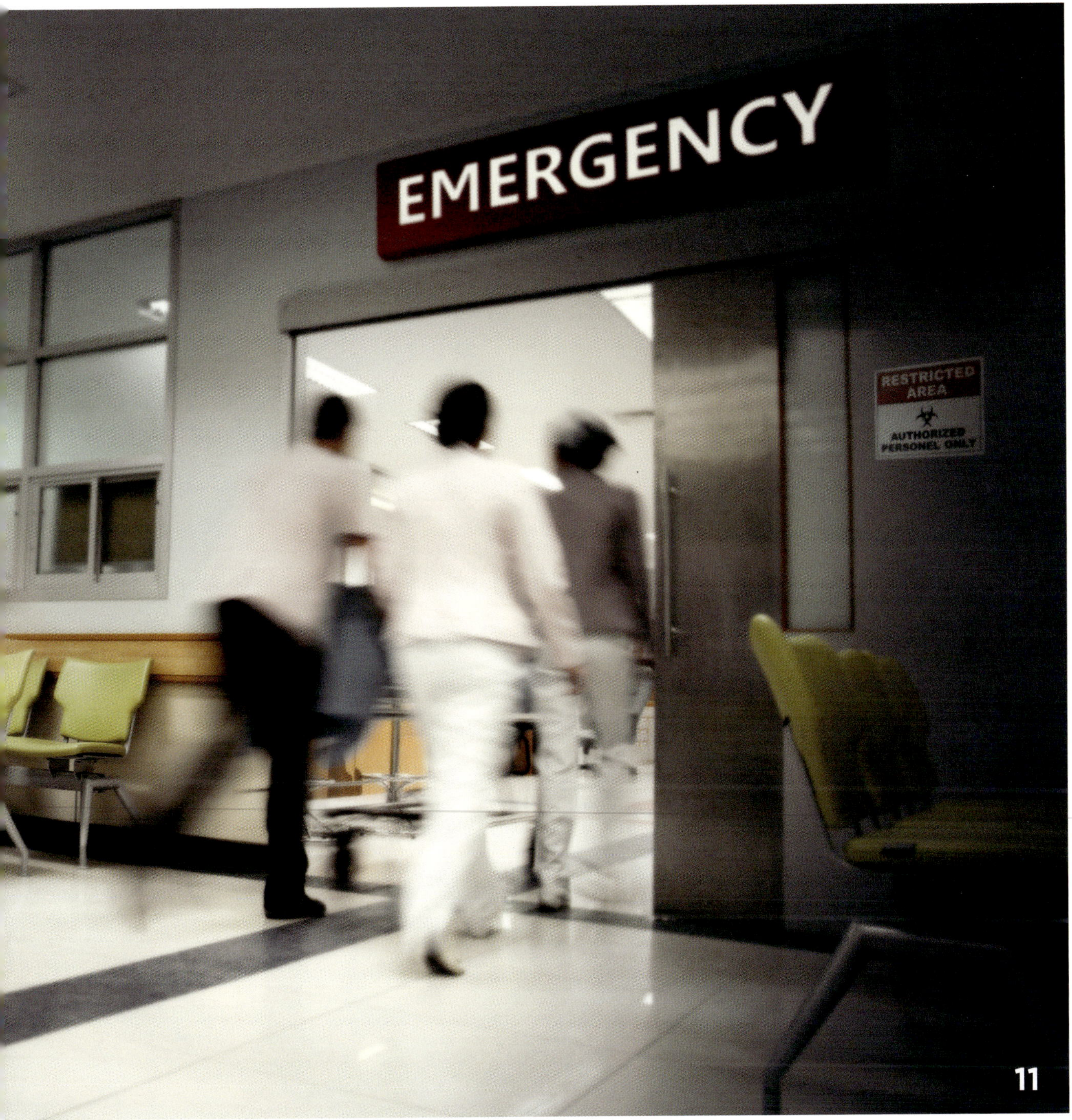
EMERGENCY
RESTRICTED AREA
AUTHORIZED PERSONEL ONLY

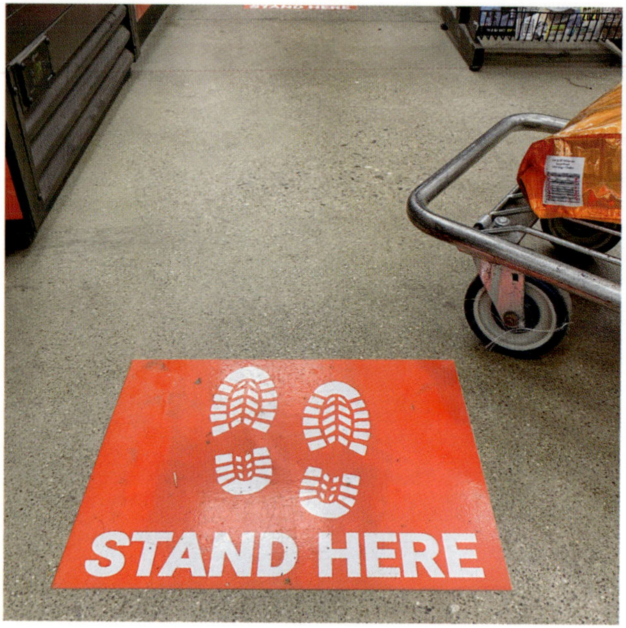

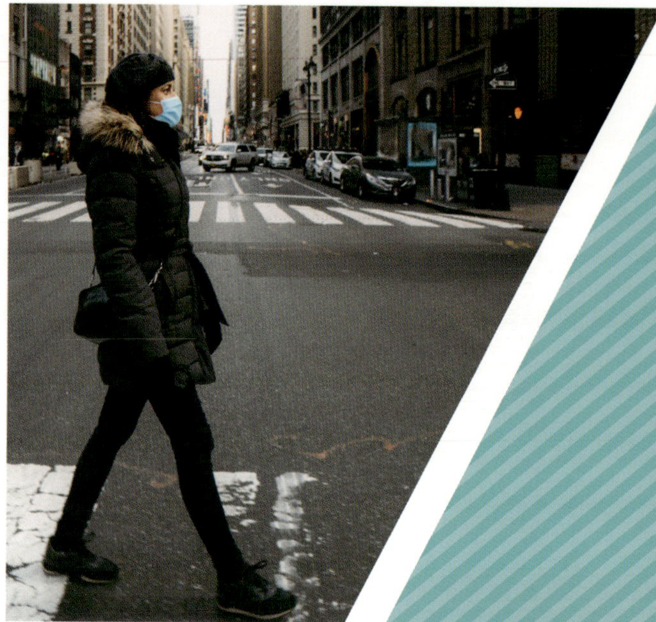

Age can also be a factor. For example, children are less affected by the coronavirus. Scientists think this might be due to their stronger immune systems.

When a pandemic occurs, the world uses emergency tools to stop the spread. Quarantine is one such tool. It forces people who are or might be infected to stay in one place. It keeps them away from others who might catch the disease. Lockdown is slightly different. It stops people from traveling.

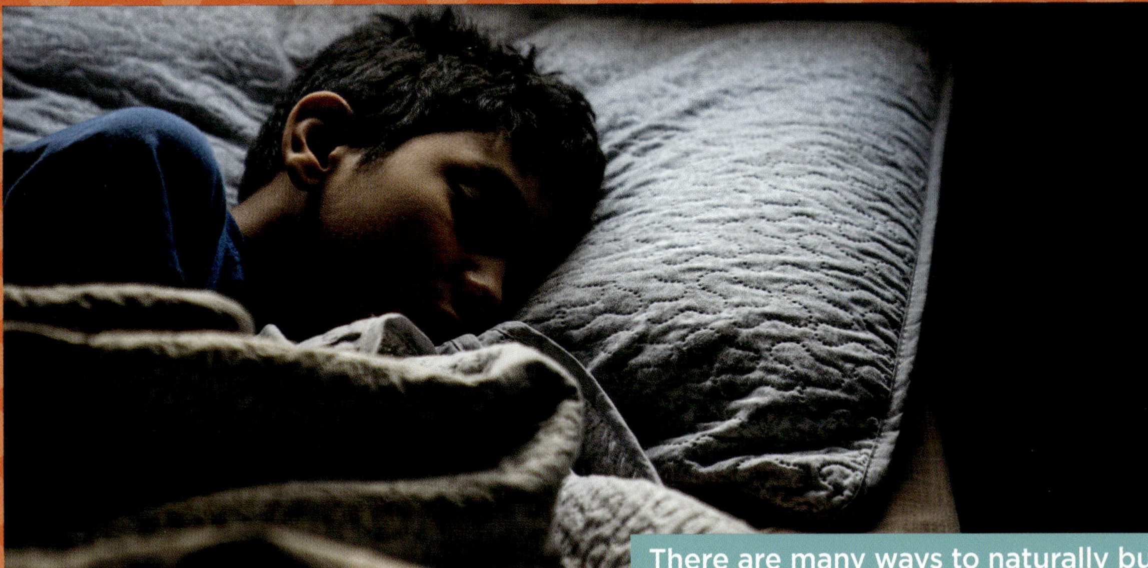

There are many ways to naturally build up and strengthen your immune system.

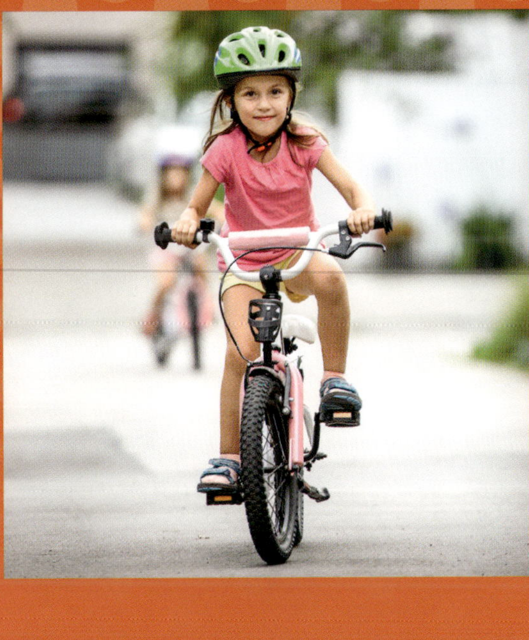

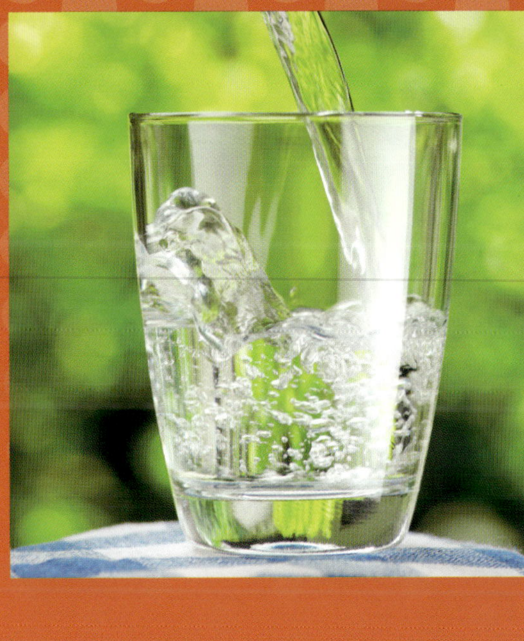

This helps keep them safe. Lockdown is normally a tool used by the government and enforced by the police. A curfew allows more movement up to a specified time of day. For example, people may be asked to stay home from 7 p.m. to 7 a.m.

Unfortunately, these tools don't always work. When many people become ill, hospitals are put under pressure. Often there aren't enough hospital beds or medications to help everyone. Hospital staff are also at risk. Doctors, nurses, and other staff can't work if they are sick.

Pandemics affect Earth too. Scientists have found that there

Think!

Think of your recent experience with COVID-19. What are the things that you have been asked to do to protect yourself and others? Why do you think it's important to be responsible and considerate of others during a pandemic?

is less noise when people are in lockdown. Transportation traffic is also reduced. This means that the air is cleaner, and there's less carbon dioxide in the atmosphere. This directly slows the effect of climate change. Animals are benefiting too. Singing birds don't have to compete with car sounds. Ocean creatures don't have to compete with noise from cruise ships.

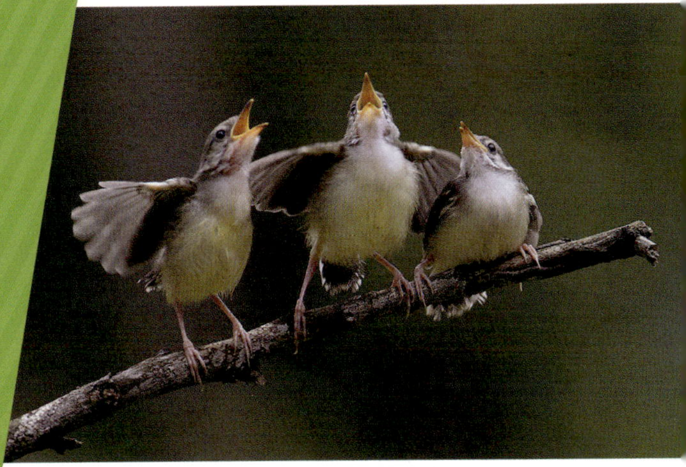

Too much noise can affect whales' stress levels.

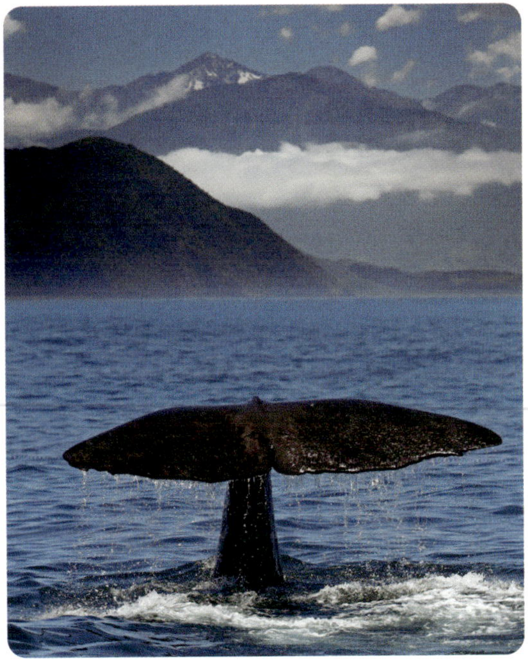

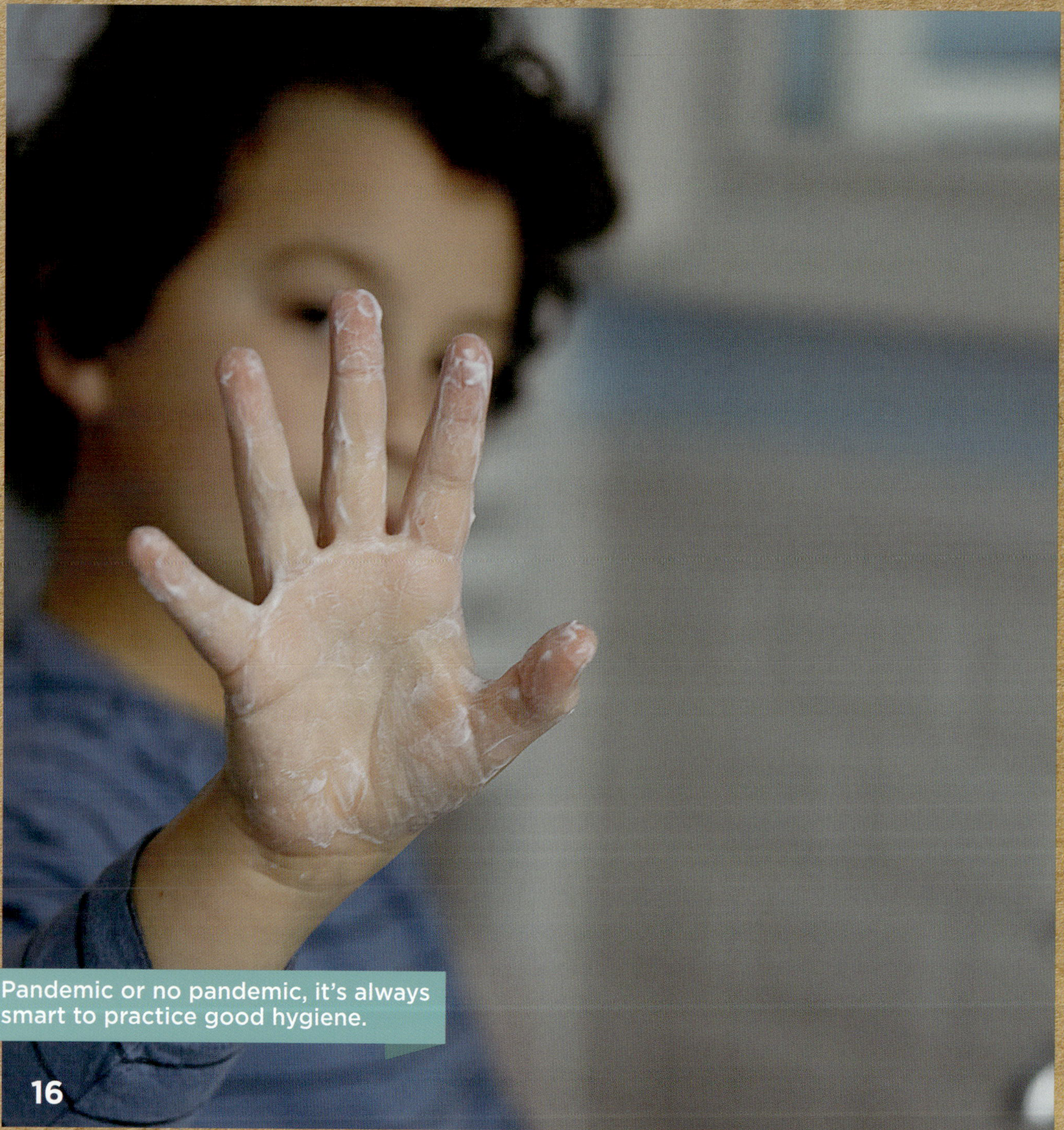

Pandemic or no pandemic, it's always smart to practice good hygiene.

PROTECTING AGAINST AND RECOVERING FROM PANDEMICS

Countries are rarely prepared for a pandemic. Each new disease is different. Some countries don't have the knowledge or funds to properly prepare. But simple rules like lockdowns or curfews can help enormously. It is important to socially distance from people during a pandemic.

Scientists play an important role in overcoming pandemics. They study the pandemic-creating diseases to find a **vaccine**. Vaccines save people's lives. Scientists worked hard to create a COVID-19 vaccine. Many of them were women. Volunteers

Look!

Everyone in the world experienced the effects of COVID-19. In many ways, the world will be forever changed. Take a look around. What's changed? Do you know a neighbor who started a mask-making business? Are you more open about talking about your feelings? Do you spend more time outdoors? Discuss this with a friend or family member.

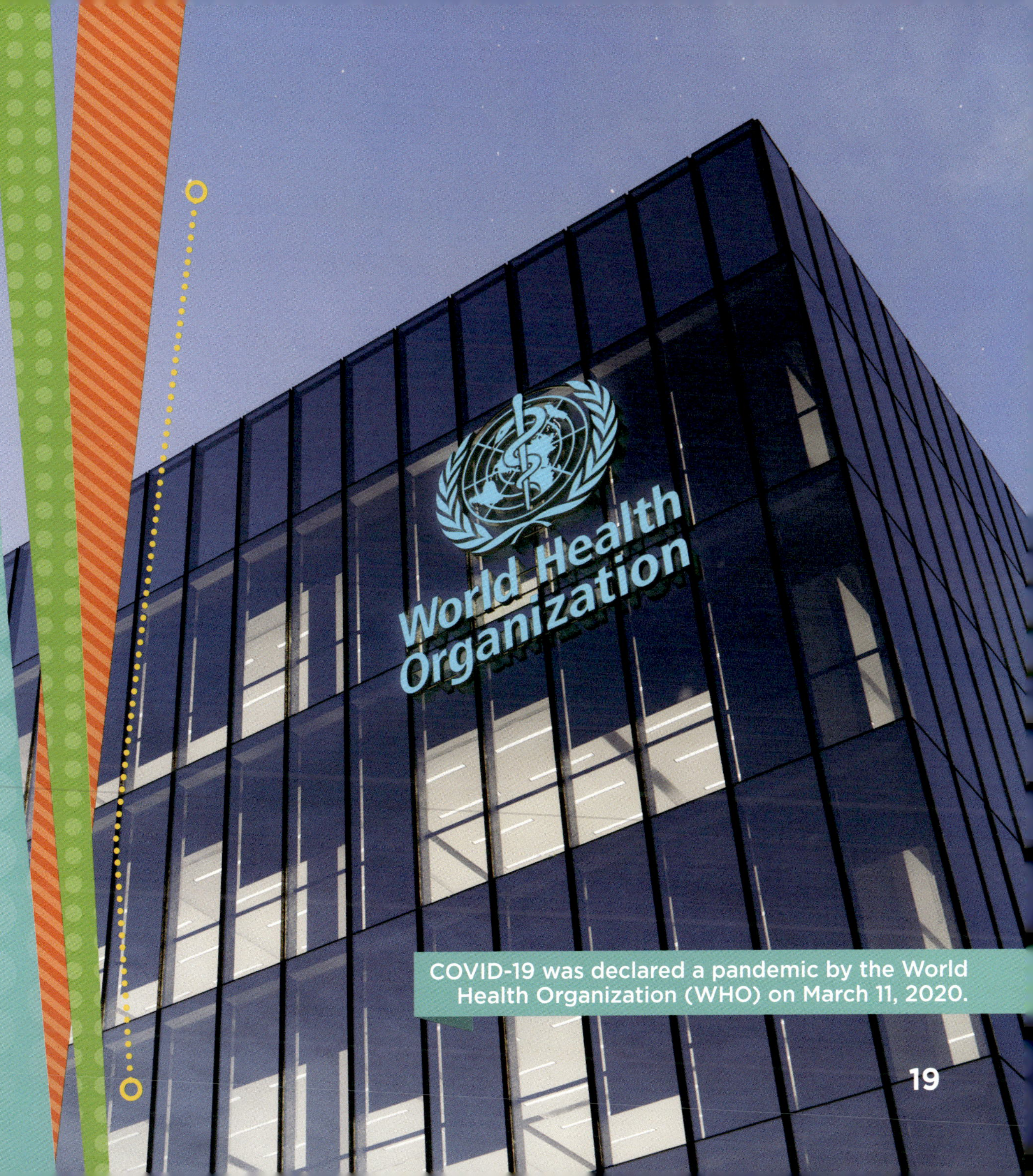

COVID-19 was declared a pandemic by the World Health Organization (WHO) on March 11, 2020.

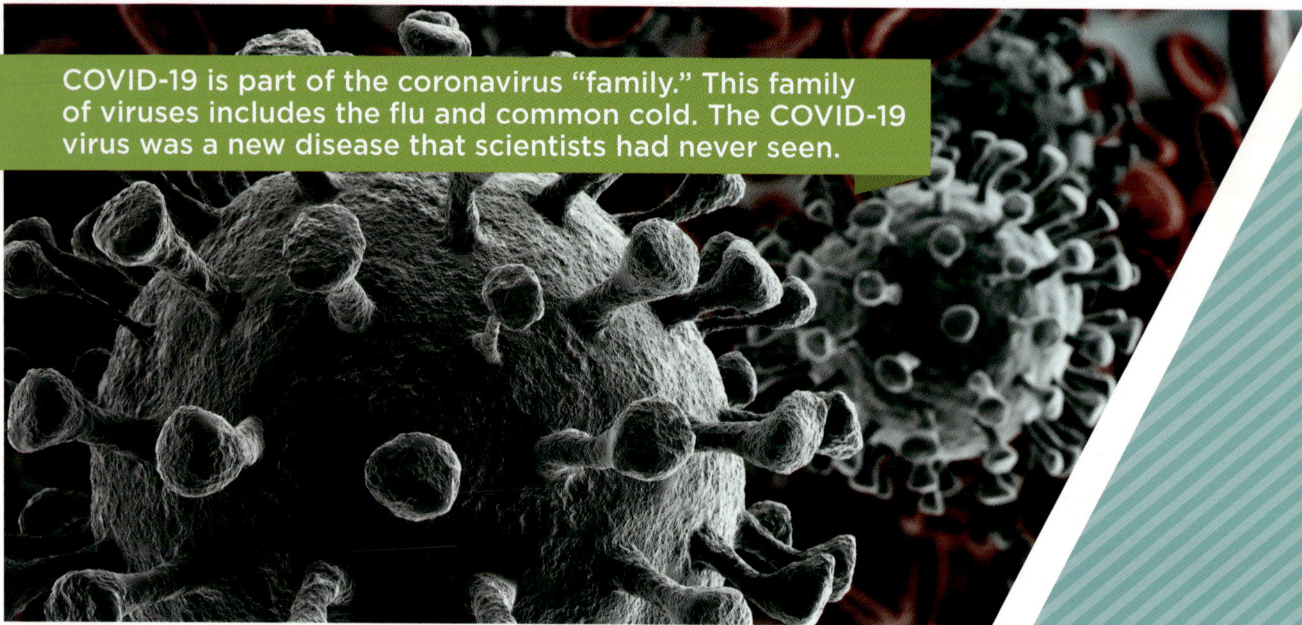

COVID-19 is part of the coronavirus "family." This family of viruses includes the flu and common cold. The COVID-19 virus was a new disease that scientists had never seen.

helped too. Scientists tested the vaccines on human volunteers to make sure that they were safe. Emergency response organizations also made sure people received help when they needed it.

Ask Questions!

Questions about mental health have been raised during the COVID-19 pandemic. People have been particularly anxious about how the lockdown has affected children. How do you think it has affected you positively and negatively?

ACTIVITY

Journaling

The COVID-19 pandemic was a scary time for everyone. One way people processed their emotions was by journaling. Sometimes writing out how you feel can help you see things in a different way. Reflecting on the positive and expressing gratitude can also help you feel better. Grab a notebook and respond to these prompts!

- How am I feeling?
- What three things am I happy about that happened today?
- What three things am I looking forward to this month?

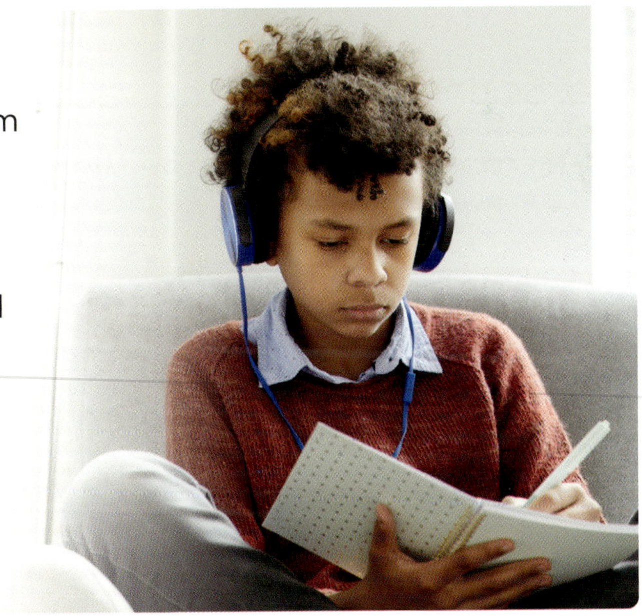

GLOSSARY

bacteria **(bak-TIHR-ee-uh)** tiny living cells; some bacteria are good for you, while others can make you sick

contagious **(kuhn-TAY-juhss)** a disease that can be spread from one person to another

dehydrated **(dee-HYE-dray-tuhd)** not having a normal amount of water in the body; dehydration makes people feel sick and can even be deadly

developing countries **(dih-VEH-luh-ping KUHN-treez)** countries with little industrial and economic activity; people in these countries generally have lower incomes than those in the developed world

epidemic **(eh-puh-DEH-mik)** a sudden increase of a disease within a particular area or country; a pandemic is a sudden increase or emergence of a disease across the entire world

immunity **(ih-MYOO-nuh-tee)** ability of the body to resist or fight a particular disease

natural disaster **(NAH-chuh-ruhl dih-ZAH-stuhr)** natural event such as a flood, earthquake, or hurricane that causes great damage

socioeconomic **(soh-see-oh-eh-kuh-NAH-mik)** used to describe the differences between groups of people, particularly their social class and financial situation

vaccine **(vak-SEEN)** a substance that is usually injected into a person or animal to protect against a particular disease

FIND OUT MORE

Books

Messner, Kate. *Plagues and Pandemics.* New York, NY: Random House Children's Books, 2021.

Stocker, Shannon. *Social Distancing.* Ann Arbor, MI: Cherry Lake Publishing, 2021.

Websites

How Pandemics Spread

https://www.youtube.com/watch?v=UG8YbNbdaco
Watch and learn how pandemics spread.

Voices from Quarantine: Kids Share Their Experiences During the Pandemic

https://www.youtube.com/watch?v=H7q04LlAvuw
Listen to kids your age talk about their experience during COVID-19.

INDEX